This Book Belongs To:

_____

_____

_____

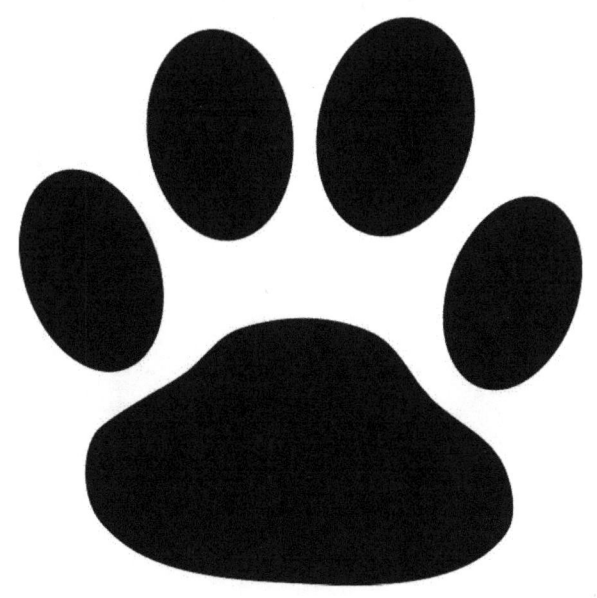

DOG RECORD BOOK

Dedication

This Dog Record Book is dedicated to all the wonderful dog people who want to track their dog's health. You are my inspiration for producing this book and I'm honored to be a part of your record keeping and the organization of your pet's health.

HOW TO USE THIS BOOK

This Dog Record Book will help you keep track of your dog's daily activities. Plus, track food intake, daily walks, vaccines and more.

Here are examples of daily tracking, checklists and prompts for you to fill in and keep records of all the details:

1. Fill In - dog and owner information, health information and behaviors

2. Track - meals and walks

3. Record - weekly notes

4. Log - Vet and Groomer appointments, medications, feeding instructions, and supplies

5. Record - vaccinations

My Dog's Personal Information

ADD PHOTO

Name	
Breed	
Color	
Date of Birth	
Spay/Neuter	
Chip ID #	
Parent Info	

Additional Information

Feeding Instructions	
Allergies Illness	
Vet Info	
Groomer Info	
Behavior Triggers	
Favorite Games	
Favorite Toys	

Meal and Walk Tracker

	AM MEAL	AM WALK	PM MEAL	PM WALK
MON				
TUES				
WED				
THUR				
FRI				
SAT				
SUN				

Weekly Notes

Veterinary Appointment	
Vaccinations	
Medication/Dosage	
Feeding Instructions	
Groomer Appointment	
Special Information	
Supplies Needed	

Meal and Walk Tracker

	AM MEAL	AM WALK	PM MEAL	PM WALK
MON				
TUES				
WED				
THUR				
FRI				
SAT				
SUN				

Weekly Notes

Veterinary Appointment	
Vaccinations	
Medication/Dosage	
Feeding Instructions	
Groomer Appointment	
Special Information	
Supplies Needed	

Meal and Walk Tracker

	AM MEAL	AM WALK	PM MEAL	PM WALK
MON				
TUES				
WED				
THUR				
FRI				
SAT				
SUN				

Weekly Notes

Veterinary Appointment	
Vaccinations	
Medication/Dosage	
Feeding Instructions	
Groomer Appointment	
Special Information	
Supplies Needed	

Meal and Walk Tracker

	AM MEAL	AM WALK	PM MEAL	PM WALK
MON				
TUES				
WED				
THUR				
FRI				
SAT				
SUN				

Weekly Notes

Veterinary Appointment	
Vaccinations	
Medication/Dosage	
Feeding Instructions	
Groomer Appointment	
Special Information	
Supplies Needed	

Meal and Walk Tracker

	AM MEAL	AM WALK	PM MEAL	PM WALK
MON				
TUES				
WED				
THUR				
FRI				
SAT				
SUN				

Weekly Notes

Veterinary Appointment	
Vaccinations	
Medication/Dosage	
Feeding Instructions	
Groomer Appointment	
Special Information	
Supplies Needed	

Meal and Walk Tracker

	AM MEAL	AM WALK	PM MEAL	PM WALK
MON				
TUES				
WED				
THUR				
FRI				
SAT				
SUN				

Weekly Notes

Veterinary Appointment	
Vaccinations	
Medication/Dosage	
Feeding Instructions	
Groomer Appointment	
Special Information	
Supplies Needed	

Meal and Walk Tracker

	AM MEAL	AM WALK	PM MEAL	PM WALK
MON				
TUES				
WED				
THUR				
FRI				
SAT				
SUN				

Weekly Notes

Veterinary Appointment	
Vaccinations	
Medication/Dosage	
Feeding Instructions	
Groomer Appointment	
Special Information	
Supplies Needed	

Meal and Walk Tracker

	AM MEAL	AM WALK	PM MEAL	PM WALK
MON				
TUES				
WED				
THUR				
FRI				
SAT				
SUN				

Weekly Notes

Veterinary Appointment	
Vaccinations	
Medication/Dosage	
Feeding Instructions	
Groomer Appointment	
Special Information	
Supplies Needed	

Meal and Walk Tracker

	AM MEAL	AM WALK	PM MEAL	PM WALK
MON				
TUES				
WED				
THUR				
FRI				
SAT				
SUN				

Weekly Notes

Veterinary Appointment	
Vaccinations	
Medication/Dosage	
Feeding Instructions	
Groomer Appointment	
Special Information	
Supplies Needed	

Meal and Walk Tracker

	AM MEAL	AM WALK	PM MEAL	PM WALK
MON				
TUES				
WED				
THUR				
FRI				
SAT				
SUN				

Weekly Notes

Veterinary Appointment	
Vaccinations	
Medication/Dosage	
Feeding Instructions	
Groomer Appointment	
Special Information	
Supplies Needed	

Meal and Walk Tracker

	AM MEAL	AM WALK	PM MEAL	PM WALK
MON				
TUES				
WED				
THUR				
FRI				
SAT				
SUN				

Weekly Notes

Veterinary Appointment	
Vaccinations	
Medication/Dosage	
Feeding Instructions	
Groomer Appointment	
Special Information	
Supplies Needed	

Meal and Walk Tracker

	AM MEAL	AM WALK	PM MEAL	PM WALK
MON				
TUES				
WED				
THUR				
FRI				
SAT				
SUN				

Weekly Notes

Veterinary Appointment	
Vaccinations	
Medication/Dosage	
Feeding Instructions	
Groomer Appointment	
Special Information	
Supplies Needed	

Meal and Walk Tracker

	AM MEAL	AM WALK	PM MEAL	PM WALK
MON				
TUES				
WED				
THUR				
FRI				
SAT				
SUN				

Weekly Notes

Veterinary Appointment	
Vaccinations	
Medication/Dosage	
Feeding Instructions	
Groomer Appointment	
Special Information	
Supplies Needed	

Meal and Walk Tracker

	AM MEAL	AM WALK	PM MEAL	PM WALK
MON				
TUES				
WED				
THUR				
FRI				
SAT				
SUN				

Weekly Notes

Veterinary Appointment	
Vaccinations	
Medication/Dosage	
Feeding Instructions	
Groomer Appointment	
Special Information	
Supplies Needed	

Meal and Walk Tracker

	AM MEAL	AM WALK	PM MEAL	PM WALK
MON				
TUES				
WED				
THUR				
FRI				
SAT				
SUN				

Weekly Notes

Veterinary Appointment	
Vaccinations	
Medication/Dosage	
Feeding Instructions	
Groomer Appointment	
Special Information	
Supplies Needed	

Meal and Walk Tracker

	AM MEAL	AM WALK	PM MEAL	PM WALK
MON				
TUES				
WED				
THUR				
FRI				
SAT				
SUN				

Weekly Notes

Veterinary Appointment	
Vaccinations	
Medication/Dosage	
Feeding Instructions	
Groomer Appointment	
Special Information	
Supplies Needed	

Meal and Walk Tracker

	AM MEAL	AM WALK	PM MEAL	PM WALK
MON				
TUES				
WED				
THUR				
FRI				
SAT				
SUN				

Weekly Notes

Veterinary Appointment	
Vaccinations	
Medication/Dosage	
Feeding Instructions	
Groomer Appointment	
Special Information	
Supplies Needed	

Meal and Walk Tracker

	AM MEAL	AM WALK	PM MEAL	PM WALK
MON				
TUES				
WED				
THUR				
FRI				
SAT				
SUN				

Weekly Notes

Veterinary Appointment	
Vaccinations	
Medication/Dosage	
Feeding Instructions	
Groomer Appointment	
Special Information	
Supplies Needed	

Meal and Walk Tracker

	AM MEAL	AM WALK	PM MEAL	PM WALK
MON				
TUES				
WED				
THUR				
FRI				
SAT				
SUN				

Weekly Notes

Veterinary Appointment	
Vaccinations	
Medication/Dosage	
Feeding Instructions	
Groomer Appointment	
Special Information	
Supplies Needed	

Meal and Walk Tracker

	AM MEAL	AM WALK	PM MEAL	PM WALK
MON				
TUES				
WED				
THUR				
FRI				
SAT				
SUN				

Weekly Notes

Veterinary Appointment	
Vaccinations	
Medication/Dosage	
Feeding Instructions	
Groomer Appointment	
Special Information	
Supplies Needed	

Meal and Walk Tracker

	AM MEAL	AM WALK	PM MEAL	PM WALK
MON				
TUES				
WED				
THUR				
FRI				
SAT				
SUN				

Weekly Notes

Veterinary Appointment	
Vaccinations	
Medication/Dosage	
Feeding Instructions	
Groomer Appointment	
Special Information	
Supplies Needed	

Meal and Walk Tracker

	AM MEAL	AM WALK	PM MEAL	PM WALK
MON				
TUES				
WED				
THUR				
FRI				
SAT				
SUN				

Weekly Notes

Veterinary Appointment	
Vaccinations	
Medication/Dosage	
Feeding Instructions	
Groomer Appointment	
Special Information	
Supplies Needed	

Meal and Walk Tracker

	AM MEAL	AM WALK	PM MEAL	PM WALK
MON				
TUES				
WED				
THUR				
FRI				
SAT				
SUN				

Weekly Notes

Veterinary Appointment	
Vaccinations	
Medication/Dosage	
Feeding Instructions	
Groomer Appointment	
Special Information	
Supplies Needed	

Meal and Walk Tracker

	AM MEAL	AM WALK	PM MEAL	PM WALK
MON				
TUES				
WED				
THUR				
FRI				
SAT				
SUN				

Weekly Notes

Veterinary Appointment	
Vaccinations	
Medication/Dosage	
Feeding Instructions	
Groomer Appointment	
Special Information	
Supplies Needed	

Meal and Walk Tracker

	AM MEAL	AM WALK	PM MEAL	PM WALK
MON				
TUES				
WED				
THUR				
FRI				
SAT				
SUN				

Weekly Notes

_____
_____
_____
_____
_____
_____
_____
_____
_____
_____
_____
_____
_____
_____
_____
_____
_____
_____
_____
_____
_____
_____
_____
_____

Veterinary Appointment	
Vaccinations	
Medication/Dosage	
Feeding Instructions	
Groomer Appointment	
Special Information	
Supplies Needed	

Meal and Walk Tracker

	AM MEAL	AM WALK	PM MEAL	PM WALK
MON				
TUES				
WED				
THUR				
FRI				
SAT				
SUN				

Weekly Notes

Veterinary Appointment	
Vaccinations	
Medication/Dosage	
Feeding Instructions	
Groomer Appointment	
Special Information	
Supplies Needed	

Meal and Walk Tracker

	AM MEAL	AM WALK	PM MEAL	PM WALK
MON				
TUES				
WED				
THUR				
FRI				
SAT				
SUN				

Weekly Notes

Veterinary Appointment	
Vaccinations	
Medication/Dosage	
Feeding Instructions	
Groomer Appointment	
Special Information	
Supplies Needed	

Meal and Walk Tracker

	AM MEAL	AM WALK	PM MEAL	PM WALK
MON				
TUES				
WED				
THUR				
FRI				
SAT				
SUN				

Weekly Notes

Veterinary Appointment	
Vaccinations	
Medication/Dosage	
Feeding Instructions	
Groomer Appointment	
Special Information	
Supplies Needed	

Meal and Walk Tracker

	AM MEAL	AM WALK	PM MEAL	PM WALK
MON				
TUES				
WED				
THUR				
FRI				
SAT				
SUN				

Weekly Notes

Veterinary Appointment	
Vaccinations	
Medication/Dosage	
Feeding Instructions	
Groomer Appointment	
Special Information	
Supplies Needed	

Meal and Walk Tracker

	AM MEAL	AM WALK	PM MEAL	PM WALK
MON				
TUES				
WED				
THUR				
FRI				
SAT				
SUN				

Weekly Notes

Veterinary Appointment	
Vaccinations	
Medication/Dosage	
Feeding Instructions	
Groomer Appointment	
Special Information	
Supplies Needed	

Meal and Walk Tracker

	AM MEAL	AM WALK	PM MEAL	PM WALK
MON				
TUES				
WED				
THUR				
FRI				
SAT				
SUN				

Weekly Notes

Veterinary Appointment	
Vaccinations	
Medication/Dosage	
Feeding Instructions	
Groomer Appointment	
Special Information	
Supplies Needed	

Meal and Walk Tracker

	AM MEAL	AM WALK	PM MEAL	PM WALK
MON				
TUES				
WED				
THUR				
FRI				
SAT				
SUN				

Weekly Notes

Veterinary Appointment	
Vaccinations	
Medication/Dosage	
Feeding Instructions	
Groomer Appointment	
Special Information	
Supplies Needed	

Meal and Walk Tracker

	AM MEAL	AM WALK	PM MEAL	PM WALK
MON				
TUES				
WED				
THUR				
FRI				
SAT				
SUN				

Weekly Notes

Veterinary Appointment	
Vaccinations	
Medication/Dosage	
Feeding Instructions	
Groomer Appointment	
Special Information	
Supplies Needed	

Meal and Walk Tracker

	AM MEAL	AM WALK	PM MEAL	PM WALK
MON				
TUES				
WED				
THUR				
FRI				
SAT				
SUN				

Weekly Notes

Veterinary Appointment	
Vaccinations	
Medication/Dosage	
Feeding Instructions	
Groomer Appointment	
Special Information	
Supplies Needed	

Meal and Walk Tracker

	AM MEAL	AM WALK	PM MEAL	PM WALK
MON				
TUES				
WED				
THUR				
FRI				
SAT				
SUN				

Weekly Notes

Veterinary Appointment	
Vaccinations	
Medication/Dosage	
Feeding Instructions	
Groomer Appointment	
Special Information	
Supplies Needed	

Meal and Walk Tracker

	AM MEAL	AM WALK	PM MEAL	PM WALK
MON				
TUES				
WED				
THUR				
FRI				
SAT				
SUN				

Weekly Notes

Veterinary Appointment	
Vaccinations	
Medication/Dosage	
Feeding Instructions	
Groomer Appointment	
Special Information	
Supplies Needed	

Meal and Walk Tracker

	AM MEAL	AM WALK	PM MEAL	PM WALK
MON				
TUES				
WED				
THUR				
FRI				
SAT				
SUN				

Weekly Notes

Veterinary Appointment	
Vaccinations	
Medication/Dosage	
Feeding Instructions	
Groomer Appointment	
Special Information	
Supplies Needed	

Meal and Walk Tracker

	AM MEAL	AM WALK	PM MEAL	PM WALK
MON				
TUES				
WED				
THUR				
FRI				
SAT				
SUN				

Weekly Notes

Veterinary Appointment	
Vaccinations	
Medication/Dosage	
Feeding Instructions	
Groomer Appointment	
Special Information	
Supplies Needed	

Meal and Walk Tracker

	AM MEAL	AM WALK	PM MEAL	PM WALK
MON				
TUES				
WED				
THUR				
FRI				
SAT				
SUN				

Weekly Notes

Veterinary Appointment	
Vaccinations	
Medication/Dosage	
Feeding Instructions	
Groomer Appointment	
Special Information	
Supplies Needed	

Meal and Walk Tracker

	AM MEAL	AM WALK	PM MEAL	PM WALK
MON				
TUES				
WED				
THUR				
FRI				
SAT				
SUN				

Weekly Notes

Veterinary Appointment	
Vaccinations	
Medication/Dosage	
Feeding Instructions	
Groomer Appointment	
Special Information	
Supplies Needed	

Meal and Walk Tracker

	AM MEAL	AM WALK	PM MEAL	PM WALK
MON				
TUES				
WED				
THUR				
FRI				
SAT				
SUN				

Weekly Notes

Veterinary Appointment	
Vaccinations	
Medication/Dosage	
Feeding Instructions	
Groomer Appointment	
Special Information	
Supplies Needed	

Meal and Walk Tracker

	AM MEAL	AM WALK	PM MEAL	PM WALK
MON				
TUES				
WED				
THUR				
FRI				
SAT				
SUN				

Weekly Notes

Veterinary Appointment	
Vaccinations	
Medication/Dosage	
Feeding Instructions	
Groomer Appointment	
Special Information	
Supplies Needed	

Meal and Walk Tracker

	AM MEAL	AM WALK	PM MEAL	PM WALK
MON				
TUES				
WED				
THUR				
FRI				
SAT				
SUN				

Weekly Notes

Veterinary Appointment	
Vaccinations	
Medication/Dosage	
Feeding Instructions	
Groomer Appointment	
Special Information	
Supplies Needed	

Meal and Walk Tracker

	AM MEAL	AM WALK	PM MEAL	PM WALK
MON				
TUES				
WED				
THUR				
FRI				
SAT				
SUN				

Weekly Notes

Veterinary Appointment	
Vaccinations	
Medication/Dosage	
Feeding Instructions	
Groomer Appointment	
Special Information	
Supplies Needed	

Meal and Walk Tracker

	AM MEAL	AM WALK	PM MEAL	PM WALK
MON				
TUES				
WED				
THUR				
FRI				
SAT				
SUN				

Weekly Notes

Veterinary Appointment	
Vaccinations	
Medication/Dosage	
Feeding Instructions	
Groomer Appointment	
Special Information	
Supplies Needed	

Meal and Walk Tracker

	AM MEAL	AM WALK	PM MEAL	PM WALK
MON				
TUES				
WED				
THUR				
FRI				
SAT				
SUN				

Weekly Notes

Veterinary Appointment	
Vaccinations	
Medication/Dosage	
Feeding Instructions	
Groomer Appointment	
Special Information	
Supplies Needed	

Meal and Walk Tracker

	AM MEAL	AM WALK	PM MEAL	PM WALK
MON				
TUES				
WED				
THUR				
FRI				
SAT				
SUN				

Weekly Notes

Veterinary Appointment	
Vaccinations	
Medication/Dosage	
Feeding Instructions	
Groomer Appointment	
Special Information	
Supplies Needed	

Meal and Walk Tracker

	AM MEAL	AM WALK	PM MEAL	PM WALK
MON				
TUES				
WED				
THUR				
FRI				
SAT				
SUN				

Weekly Notes

Veterinary Appointment	
Vaccinations	
Medication/Dosage	
Feeding Instructions	
Groomer Appointment	
Special Information	
Supplies Needed	

Meal and Walk Tracker

	AM MEAL	AM WALK	PM MEAL	PM WALK
MON				
TUES				
WED				
THUR				
FRI				
SAT				
SUN				

Weekly Notes

Veterinary Appointment	
Vaccinations	
Medication/Dosage	
Feeding Instructions	
Groomer Appointment	
Special Information	
Supplies Needed	

Meal and Walk Tracker

	AM MEAL	AM WALK	PM MEAL	PM WALK
MON				
TUES				
WED				
THUR				
FRI				
SAT				
SUN				

Weekly Notes

Veterinary Appointment	
Vaccinations	
Medication/Dosage	
Feeding Instructions	
Groomer Appointment	
Special Information	
Supplies Needed	

Meal and Walk Tracker

	AM MEAL	AM WALK	PM MEAL	PM WALK
MON				
TUES				
WED				
THUR				
FRI				
SAT				
SUN				

Weekly Notes

Veterinary Appointment	
Vaccinations	
Medication/Dosage	
Feeding Instructions	
Groomer Appointment	
Special Information	
Supplies Needed	

Meal and Walk Tracker

	AM MEAL	AM WALK	PM MEAL	PM WALK
MON				
TUES				
WED				
THUR				
FRI				
SAT				
SUN				

Weekly Notes

Veterinary Appointment	
Vaccinations	
Medication/Dosage	
Feeding Instructions	
Groomer Appointment	
Special Information	
Supplies Needed	

Vaccinations

Date	Vaccination	Given By	Age	Next Due

Vaccinations

Date	Vaccination	Given By	Age	Next Due

Vaccinations

Date	Vaccination	Given By	Age	Next Due

Vaccinations

Date	Vaccination	Given By	Age	Next Due

Vaccinations

Date	Vaccination	Given By	Age	Next Due

www.ingramcontent.com/pod-product-compliance
Lightning Source LLC
Chambersburg PA
CBHW080811040426

42333CB00062B/2687